Pierre KITHA BITINGO LUSAMBIA
Félix ATADOKPEDE

EPIDEMIOLOGICAL, CLINICAL AND THERAPEUTIC ASPECTS OF ERYTHEMA PIGMENTOSA

Pierre KITHA BITINGO LUSAMBIA
Félix ATADOKPEDE

EPIDEMIOLOGICAL, CLINICAL AND THERAPEUTIC ASPECTS OF ERYTHEMA PIGMENTOSA

Multicenter study

ScienciaScripts

Imprint

Cover image: www.ingimage.com

This book is a translation from the original published under ISBN 978-620-8-82459-4.

Publisher:
Sciencia Scripts
is a trademark of
Dodo Books Indian Ocean Ltd. and OmniScriptum S.R.L publishing group

120 High Road, East Finchley, London, N2 9ED, United Kingdom
Str. Armeneasca 28/1, office 1, Chisinau MD-2012, Republic of Moldova, Europe
Managing Directors: Ieva Konstantinova, Victoria Ursu
info@omniscriptum.com

Printed at: see last page
ISBN: 978-620-8-99083-1

IN MEMORIAM

- To the memory of my parents **Joseph Bitingo Lusambia Lukabia and Elisabeth Mpala Kyamonakombe and my older brother André Bitingo**, you left us at a very young age, your series of departures made me disgusted with life, but thanks to the Lord, I can hold on again. You have your place in my heart, dad, mum and big brother. I feel ambivalent, between sadness and joy, because this end of my training would be for you the realisation of what you have sown and planted in me for several years by showing me the way to school. I'm crying but I know that you're alive and you'll always be by my side.

- In memory of our late **Master Hubert YEDOMON**, Professor of Dermatology and Venereology, may God grant you a peaceful and eternal rest.

DEDICACES

- To my father **Joseph Bitingo Lusambia Lukabia**, this work is the fruit of your initiative to see me continue my studies, by reminding me of this phrase, son, you have finished general medicine, I want you to start specialisation. You have consented to my education. May God grant you eternal rest with him, Dad. I would love to see you by my side at this time.

- To my mother **Elisabeth Mpala Kyamonakombe**, who bore me in her womb. I dedicate this work to you. May Almighty God grant you eternal rest in his presence. I dedicate this work to you, my dear mother, for my first steps at school and also your lessons on our blackboard, you knew how to repeat the lessons learned and anticipate future ones in spite of your tasks. Mum, words fail me. My love for you is eternal.

- To my late big **brother André Bitingo Kantalingi**, my homo doctor. Your departure was unexpected and put an end to our joint projects. You have left a void in my heart, big brother. May the Lord grant you eternal rest.

- To my sisters and brothers **Dina Mpala Bitingo, Sylvie Fatouma Bitingo, Jacques Bitingo Busaga and Antoine Bitingo Wasolela**, my precious gifts from God, it is a grace for me to be born among you. You have been with me on all fronts of my training and you have taken care of it properly, your finances have never forgotten me and you have provided financially and morally for my training stay. I dedicate this work to all of you to show my gratitude to all of you, my co-workers, I love you all.
- To our brother-in-law **Jules Mastaki Safari**, your love is no longer a secret. You were one of the pioneers of this training project.

- To my sweetheart **Angel Nkomba Ngossa**, thank you for your support, your prayers and your gentle words of encouragement.

- **To my sisters-in-law, Rachelle Fatouma and Aziza Lehani Afie**, your support for me goes without saying. I would like to call you the pillars of the family. No family can prosper without a balanced husband and wife. Thank you for the peace you bring to your couples.

- To my nephews, nieces and cousins, **Beni Mugisho Nyalulerha, Elisabeth Safari Wani, Marcelline Safari Munyerenkana, Albertine Mawamini Safari, Quernas Safari Mastaki and Christelle Bitingo Kantalingi**, your support has been considerable and of great importance in making this project a reality. I love you all.

ACKNOWLEDGEMENTS

I would like to take this solemn opportunity to express my sincere thanks and gratitude:

- **To Professor Emeritus Florencia do ANGO-PADONOU**, it is a great honour that you have given us access to training.

- To **our dissertation supervisor Professor Félix ATADOKPEDE**, your love of work, your concern to pass on knowledge until your learners' ignorance is overcome, your knowledge, your orthodoxy, your simplicity and your paternal sense have aroused our admiration throughout our training.

- **To Professor Hugues ADEGBIDI**, your paternal love and your simplicity are qualities that will remain engraved in our memory.

- **To Professor Christiane KOUDOUKPO**, your scientific rigour, your simplicity and your human and social qualities make you more than a teacher, they make you a mother. We will never forget your encouragement at the beginning of each session, which gave us hope of finishing the course.

- **To Maitre de Conférences Agrégée Bérénice DEGBOE**, your rigour and sense of perfection have left a deep impression on us. Your concern to empathise with others has also left its mark on us, and we have found in you a mother who is more than just a teacher.

- **To Associate Professor Fabrice AKPADJAN**, your method of self-discovery has left a deep impression on us. When it came to making ourselves understood, we were never in a hurry until the person to whom the question was addressed managed to find the answer on their own. This approach has left a lasting impression on us, and we'll be using it when we're as good as you are.

- To **Associate Professor Nadège AGBESSI**, your encouragement and exhortation to work have left a deep impression on us.

- To my elder doctors, **Alida KOUASSI, Odile HOUNGBO, Nadège ELEGBEDE, Nina MAFFO and Serge OTEME, Gloria NOUHOUMON, Aline WAPI, Sintia KOUNKOU, Armelle TAZANOU**, thank you for your support and encouragement, not forgetting your patience in helping us to understand things.

- To my dear colleagues **Edson Adégbidi, Sylvaine Pentoue, Diane Assogba and Dahlia Tounouga**, reminding me of our first days of probation until today. I'd like to take the liberty of calling you valiant heroes. I'd like to thank you for having written a story of my life with you, and you are sealed in my heart forever. Not everything was rosy, but we knew how to manage our differences as adults. Thank you for putting up with my weaknesses.

- To the DES Dermatology-Venerology doctors, **Dahlia Tounouga, Cordule Balola, Marie-Christelle Legonou, Laura Dotsop, Boubacar Mahaman, Florys Mastaki, Blandine Omono, Pascal Bisimwa, Marielle Ayinadou, Nadia Ntouala, Yeouna Ndembi, Marielle Ragi Lya Lushule, Fleurine Leukelem, Sophie Remadji, Marlyse Hounyeme, Fabienne Adandenjan, Guylain Nzanzu**, thank you for all the good times we had together.

- To all our lecturers at the Bamako Dermatology Hospital, **Professor Ousmane Faye, Maître de Conférences Agrégé Adama Aguissa Dicko, Maître de Conférences Agrégé Mamadou Gassama Dr Binta Guindo, Dr Yamoussa Karabinta, Dr Cissé Lamissa, Dr Bekaye Traoré, Dr Madou Sissoko, Dr Alimata Keita, Dr Koureissi Tall**. Thank you for your availability, guidance and welcome to the Bamako Dermatology Hospital.

- To my DES colleagues in Bamako, in particular **Maimouna Diallo, Djeneba Koné, Djeneba Keita, Ismaila Bamba and Promoubé Kamaté**, a sincere thank you for the good times we had together.

- To all the paramedical staff at the **CUDEV**, the **CDTUB-Allada** and the **CMP**, I'm delighted to have been one of you, and I'd like to thank you for the good collaboration and for everything you taught me.

- To my brothers **Anato Zinsou Paul, Tenkou Jérémie, Mbuya Musapudi Erick, Kahenga Victor, Kabaya Kashombo Jean Guy, Fokoua Fogno Cyrille Osée**. Your wise advice and support are invaluable. You made my stay in Cotonou a pleasant one.

- To all those who have contributed in any way to the realisation of this work, my deepest gratitude. To all those whose names are not forgotten, thank you for your support and encouragement. I pray to God that our friendship and fraternity will be eternal.

INTRODUCTION

Erythema pigmentum fixans (EPF) is an adverse skin reaction characterised by the appearance of a rash at a fixed site on the body each time a specific drug is ingested. The number of sites may increase with each recurrence. The lesions may be covered with vesicles and/or bullae, in which case it is called bullous EPF, and when they cover a large body surface area, the rash is called generalised bullous fixed erythema pigmentosa (GBFPE). Because of the generalised skin denudation that can be seen in this condition, GBPE can be confused clinically with Stevens-Johnson syndrome/toxic epidermal necrolysis (SJS/NET)[1] .

More than 100 drugs are currently implicated. Erythema pigmentum is typically drug-induced[2] . However, rare cases of dietary causes have been reported[3] . The main inducing drugs are analgesics (pyrazoles, paracetamol, aspirin), antibiotics (sulphonamides, cyclins), anti-epileptics (phenytoin, barbiturates, carbamazepine) and NSAIDs[4] . The pigmentary sequelae of this toxidermia make it possible to make a retrospective diagnosis. There are several clinical forms. EPFBG is the most severe form, making EPF both a benign and a severe form of toxidermia. The positive diagnosis appears easy, as opposed to the aetiological diagnosis, which requires a more or less complex methodical approach. Treatment remains symptomatic. Prevention consists of avoiding the drug in question by drawing up a drug allergy avoidance card. Today, it is estimated that drug-induced hyperpigmentation accounts for 20% of all cases of acquired hyperpigmentation .[5]

In sub-Saharan Africa, few studies have addressed this issue. *Yoboué et al* in 2005 in Côte d'Ivoire found that EPF accounted for 84.55% of the chemical causes of dyschromia[5] . Studies on the epidemiological and clinical aspects, such as our own, were carried out by Atadokpèdé and Saka in Benin and Togo in 2009 and 2012 respectively.

In Latin America, EPF generally occurs after exposure to antiepileptic drugs such as carbamazepine in several studies, including that of *Veronica et al.* in Colombia in 2006[6] . The lack of recent epidemiological, clinical and therapeutic data was our motivation for initiating this study.

General objective

To study the epidemiological, clinical and therapeutic aspects of EPF at the CUDEV, the CMP and the CDTUB in Allada.

Specific objectives

- To determine the prevalence of erythema pigmentum fixata at CUDEV, CMP and the Dermatology-Venerology Department of the CDTUB in Allada.
- Describe the clinical characteristics of EPF at the CUDEV, the CMP and the Dermatology-Venerology Department of the CDTUB-Allada.
- Describe the therapeutic characteristics of EPF at the CUDEV, the CMP and the Dermatology and Venereology Department of the CDTUB-Allada.
- Identify the drugs responsible for EPF at the CUDEV, the CMP and the Dermatology-Venerology Department of the CDTUB-Allada

1. GENERAL

1.1. Definition

Fixed erythema pigmentosum (FEP) is an acute drug reaction characterised by the appearance of macular lesions, sometimes topped by bullae, which may affect the skin and mucous membranes, and which occur at the same sites when the inducing drug is re-exposed.

1.2 Interest

- Epidemiology: EPF is a ubiquitous toxidermia, affecting all breeds without distinction.
- Diagnosis: the diagnosis is clinical
- Therapeutics: avoidance of the compound in question and its relatives is the cornerstone of treatment,
- Prognosis: pigmentary sequelae are the cosmetic complication of this condition.

1.3. History

Pathognomonic of toxidermia, it is the only dermatosis caused exclusively by drugs. It consists of a few (1 to 10) rounded erythematous plaques, a few centimetres in diameter, often painful and infiltrated (Figure 4). They may be covered by a bulla. The concept of erythema pigmentum fixata (EPF) was introduced by Brocq in 1894. It begins within hours (< 48 hours) of the inducing drug being taken.

Fixed food eruption (FFE) is a clinical entity first described in 1992 by Haztis following ingestion of cheese crisps .[7,8]

1.4. Epidemiology

The incidence of EPF has not been established. Within toxidermia, the frequency of EPF varies considerably from one continent to another, and within the same continent from one country to another: in Asia, EPF accounts for between 11% and 30% of all toxidermias in Indian series, 15.3% in a retrospective Chinese series [4], and 9% in a prospective Thai series. EPF is a widely reported toxidermia in Pakistan and Turkey[1 1,12].

In Africa, on dark skin, these lesions appear as hyperpigmented macules with erythematous borders and clear boundaries . [11]

A few years ago, anti-infective sulphonamides were the main cause of EPF[12] . Today, the trend has changed and any drug is likely to induce EPF, not forgetting certain foods. This is the case with anti-histamines, which have been fingered several times since 2000 . [13–15]

In Europe, EPF is considered to be rare. Allergological investigation of EPF has moved up a gear with the introduction of the FISARD group method. Patch testing performed in situ on the site previously affected by EPF is an interesting way of investigating this toxidermia. If in situ patch tests are negative, it may be useful to carry out repeated application tests (ROAT test) on the site previously affected by EPF. Few studies have reported on the sensitivity of patch tests and repeated application tests . [9,16]

In Asia, as in Africa, EPF remains a common toxidermia. These geographical differences may be partly explained by a possible genetic predisposition, which has not yet been fully explored in this type of toxidermia .[17,18]

1.5. Pathophysiology

Erythema pigmentum fixans (EPF) is a model of delayed drug hypersensitivity mediated by CD8 T lymphocytes (LT). The positivity of patch tests in the investigation of these eruptions also supports this hypothesis [27]. However, the rapid onset of the reaction (within hours of administration) makes this an atypical model.

Intra-epidermal CD8 LTs play a major role in the development of the disease. In EPF lesions, these LT have an "effector" phenotype . [9]

Fixed erythema pigmentum (FPE) is due to a localised cytotoxic reaction by CD8+ T lymphocytes, leading to activation and damage to keratinocytes expressing intercellular adhesion molecule (ICAM) 1 (CD54). This T cell activation is prolonged but remains localised.

- The absence of widespread lesions could be due to immune regulation by CD4+ T lymphocytes.
- The cytokines released by activated keratinocytes lead to autocrine amplification of neighbouring keratinocytes and antigen-independent stimulation of cytotoxic lymphocytes .[19,20]

The pathophysiological hypothesis of toxidermia postulates that mild and severe forms obey the same mechanisms and that they are a spectrum of drug-specific activation of cytotoxic CD8+ T lymphocytes. Individuals are sensitised in lymphoid organs by interaction between dendritic cells (DC) and T lymphocytes (TL). This DC/TL interaction involves the production and clonal proliferation of cytotoxic CD8+ T cells (purple), which cause toxidermia, and regulatory CD4+ T cells with anti-inflammatory activity, which block the functions of CD8+ T cells. When the drug is reintroduced, CD4+ and CD8+ LT are recruited and activated in the skin due to the expression of peptide/drug complexes by skin cells. The CD8+ LT recruited are heterogeneous and made up of numerous clones with different functions. Few CD8+ LT are terminally differentiated and therefore capable of producing the full range of cytotoxic mechanisms. Keratinocytes express MHC class I molecules and are therefore capable of activating cytotoxic CD8+ LT which induce apoptosis/necrosis of keratinocytes. Dendritic cells and macrophages express MHC class II molecules and activate LT regulators. This balance between epidermal damage induced by CD8+ LT and the anti-inflammatory effect of CD4+ LT concerns a moderate and regulated cutaneous inflammation which is also composed of NK cells, monocytes and polynuclear cells . [21]

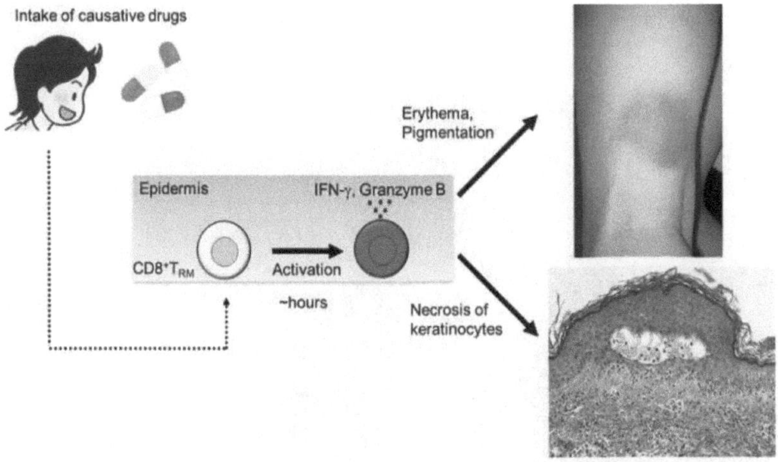

Figure1 : Pathophysiology of EPF. Yoshiki et al. Japan. 2021.

1.6 Clinical study

EPF can take on a variety of clinical presentations, ranging from a single pigmented lesion to more extensive bullous lesions, normopigmented EPF or even pseudo-Lyell's syndrome, without the cause or pathophysiology being different. The onset of this toxidermia is relatively short, ranging from a few days to 2 weeks. This period may be reduced to a few hours when the offending compound is reintroduced.[9,22]

1.6.1. Type of description: Fixed erythema pigmentosum in its common form

Skin and mucous membrane lesions.

- **Clinical signs**

Functional sign: pruritus and/or tingling

General signs: none

Physical signs: rounded erythematous plaques (1 to 10), 2 to 5 centimetres in diameter, often painful and infiltrated. Located symmetrically on the trunk and limbs. The mucous membranes of the mouth and anogenital area are frequently affected.

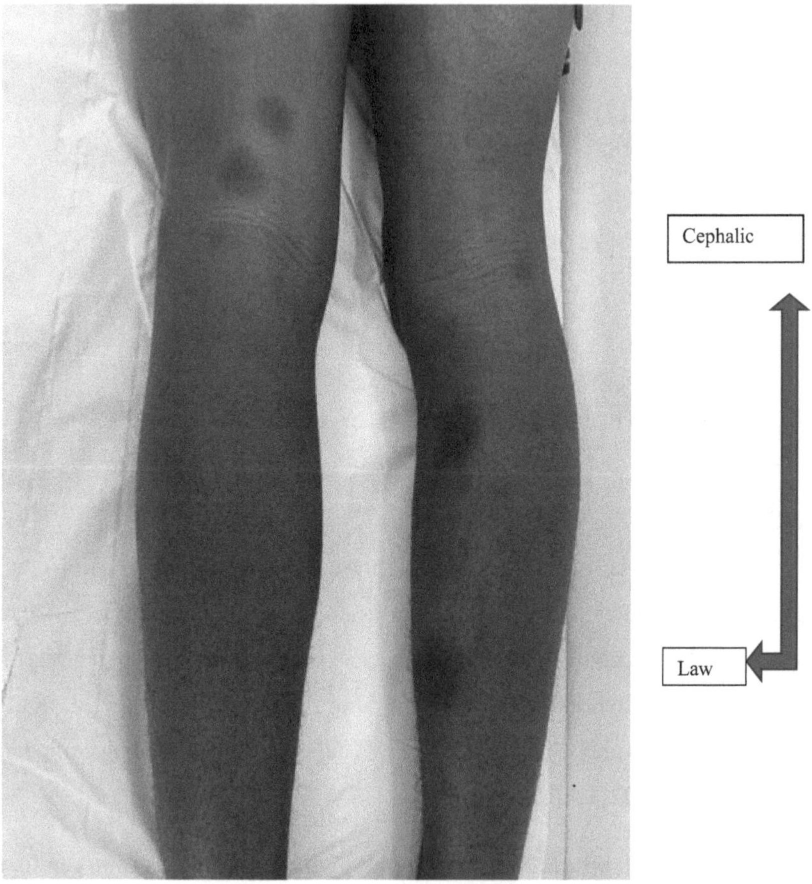

Figure2 : EPF hyperpigmented macules (Photo CUDEV June 2021)

- **Paraclinical examinations**
    - **Histopathology**

Histopathological examination typically reveals keratinocytic necrosis, sometimes confluent, which may be responsible for subepidermal detachment. The mononuclear infiltrate is often more abundant than in NET, affecting the superficial and deep dermis. It is associated with lymphocytes, eosinophilic polynuclear cells and sometimes neutrophils of interstitial but also perivascular topography. In recurrent forms, melanophages accumulate in the dermis.[9,10]

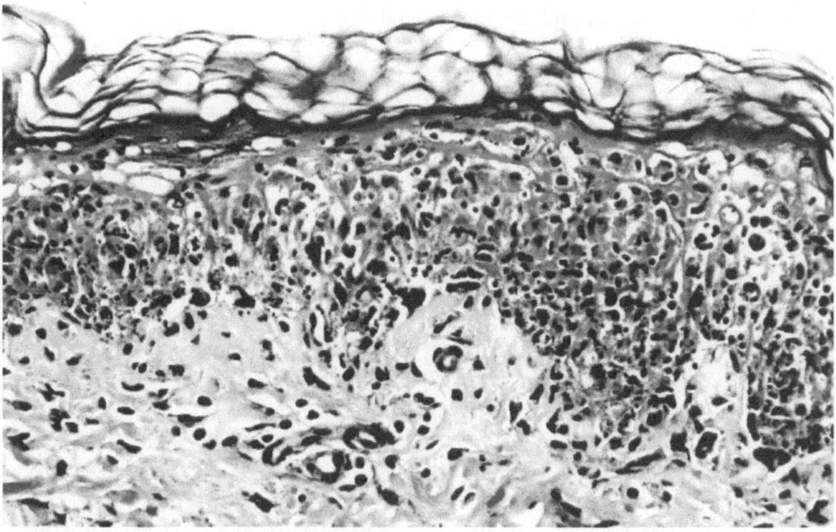

Figure3 : histopathological image of erythema pigmentosum fixans. Weyers W, Metze et al D. Dermatol Pract Concept. 31 Jan 2011.

- **Allergy tests**

Erythema pigmentum fixans (EPF) is a non-severe toxidermia, except in the case of a generalised bullous form (EPFBG). Once the lesions have healed, the drug-specific memory T lymphocytes remain strictly localised to the mucocutaneous areas affected by EPF; in situ patch tests (*PTis*) or repeated open application in situ tests (*ROATis*) are therefore recommended. If these tests are negative, with the exception of EPFBG, a provocation test (PT) can be used to confirm the responsibility of a drug.

1.6.2. Clinical forms

1.6.2.1. Morphological forms

- **Generalized fixed bullous erythema pigmentosum**

Erythema pigmentosum bullosum generalis (EPFBG) is a potentially fatal form of severe toxidermia in elderly patients. Commonly used drugs such as analgesics (NSAIDs, paracetamol) and antibiotics (penicillins) are frequently responsible. EPFBG is a serious, even lethal, toxidermia caused by a skin failure syndrome in elderly patients. If diagnosed, precessive episodes can identify the drug responsible. Medication errors are common in this fragile population. Self-medication, particularly with painkillers, is widespread. Paracetamol, a classic inducer of EPFBG, is often not considered to be a drug, let alone a contraindication. Memory problems and the multiplicity of generics can increase the risk of a repeat of a previous culprit. As for penicillins, they may be prescribed incorrectly because the severity of the allergy declared is not known or underestimated. These cases have occurred despite correct information being given to the patient and his or her family, and a record being made in the patient's computer file. Allergy alert systems need to be optimised. Increased vigilance is required in the case of elderly patients, for whom these serious, even fatal, toxidermias are sometimes avoidable .[9,23]

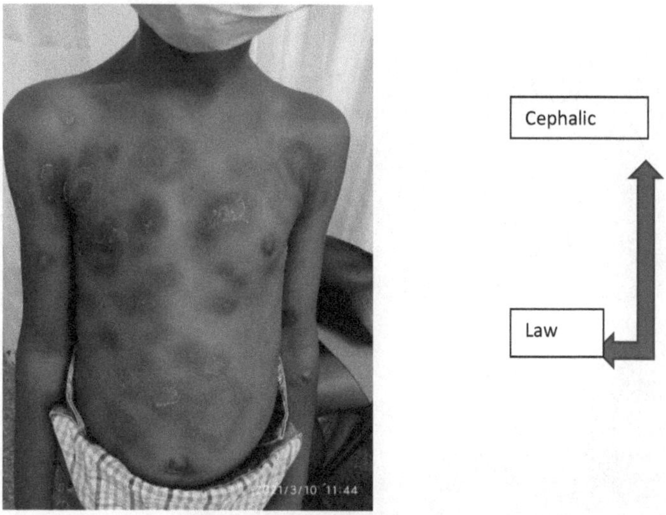

Figure4 : Bullous EPF attributable to paracetamol in a 10-year-old child, HDB. May 2024

- **Localised fixed bullous erythema pigmentosa**

EPFBL is a toxidermia requiring specialised management. It is a model of delayed hypersensitivity to drugs mediated by TCD8+ lymphocytes. It affects all parts of the body, but in the majority of cases is confined to the mucous membranes. Involvement of the genital mucosa is rare. EPFBL is more commonly found in males, with a preferential location in the glans penis and balanopreputial fold. It poses a diagnostic problem when it occurs in isolation, along with pemphigus, genital herpes and erythema multiforme major, which is why it is so important to carry out a thorough history-taking to check for previous drug use .[24]

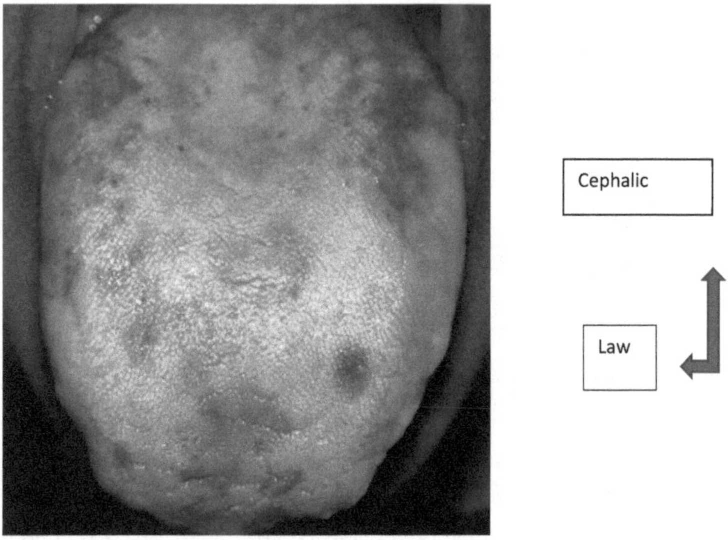

Figure5 : Fixed erythema pigmentosa of the buccal mucosa attributable to zidovudine. Photo Lotfi. 2022

- **Non-pigmented or normopigmented fixed erythema pigmentosa**

There are forms of EPF with no pigmentary sequelae. This is paradoxical in relation to the natural history of the disease, which develops into pigmentary incontinence, responsible for the residual pigmentation of the disease. It is difficult to diagnose. The appearance of lesions at the same site in a context of drug use, after thorough questioning, provides diagnostic support . [25]

1.6.2.2. Topographical shapes

- **Fixed erythema pigmentosum of the genital mucosa**

They are generally found on the lips, genitals and penis in men. The eruptions generally occur within a few hours of administration of the drug and disappear spontaneously. This clinical form poses a diagnostic problem in conjunction with herpetic recurrence and other dermatoses affecting the mucous membranes, such as atrophic lichen sclerosus or autoimmune pemphigus.

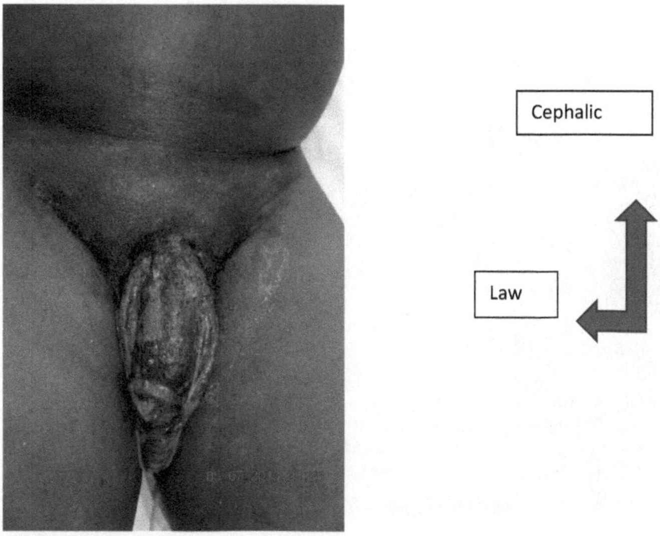

Figure6 : Bullous EPF in the erosive stage of male OGE. CUDEV. April 2024

1.6.2.3. Forms by age

Erythema pigmentum multiforme in children

Erythema pigmentum fixans (EPF) is a benign toxidermia, and its clinical features in children are identical to those in adults. However, the presence of EPF in children can lead to confusion with café au lait spots in genodermatoses such as Von Recklinghausen's disease.

It initially manifests itself as one or more rounded or oval, erythematous or purplish macules that are very well defined, sometimes developing into bullae, and are stinging rather than pruritic. The lesions may be single or multiple and may affect the skin or, more rarely, the mucous membranes .[26]

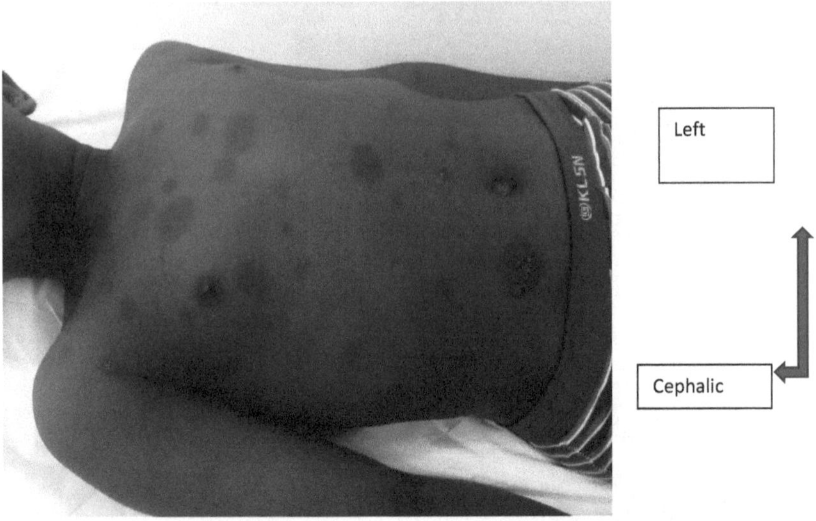

Figure7 : Fixed erythema pigmentosum in children. CUDEV, November 2023

- **Erythema pigmentosa associated with HIV infection**

EPF is a toxidermia commonly encountered in HIV-positive patients. The occurrence of EPF in a single patient with different molecules is often a circumstance in the discovery of HIV infection. For a long time, antiretroviral therapy was blamed for EPF around the time of its introduction. The clinical manifestations are the same as in uninfected subjects [27]

- **Fixed erythema pigmentosa associated with autoimmune diseases**

Autoimmune diseases are among the risk factors for EPF because of the heavy therapy they require, but also because of immune abnormalities. This could be explained by the hypothesis of certain toxidermias and certain genotypes of the HLA system . [28]

1.6.3.4. Evolution of fixed erythema pigmentosa

Erythema pigmentum fixans is a spectrum toxidermia that can develop benignly or be complicated by major toxidermia.

EPF is characterised by rapid healing following discontinuation of the compound, leaving residual pigmentation. If the offending drug is reintroduced, the rash recurs much more quickly. Lesions typically recur in the same places, but may also be more numerous, or even be associated with a higher proportion of bullous lesions . [9,11,29]

These lesions may be covered by a bulla (bullous EPF). The inflammatory lesions disappear within a few days, leaving brown or slate-coloured pigmented patches. If the inducing drug is reintroduced, the lesions recur at the same site and may often spread to new areas. Reintroduction may lead to the development of a severe bullous form of EPF.

1.7 Diagnosis

1.7.1. Positive diagnosis

Epidemiological argument: the patient may have taken medication when the lesions appeared.

Clinical argument: the diagnosis is often clinical. It is based on well-directed and often police questioning and a physical examination revealing rounded erythematous plaques, 2 to 5 centimetres in diameter, often painful and infiltrated, located symmetrically on the trunk and limbs. The oral and anogenital mucosa are frequently affected. Lesions recur at the same site and can often spread to new areas.

Paraclinical evidence: patch tests may be used, as well as dermatopathology in rare cases.

1.7.2. Differential diagnosis

- In the localised form, the main differential diagnosis is spider bites, or even a reaction to insect bites such as prurigo strophulus.
- In the form with genital involvement, herpetic recurrence and lichen sclero-atrophic.
- In bullous forms, toxic epidermal necrolysis (TEN), erythema multiforme and autoimmune bullous dermatoses (Ig A linear dermatosis, pemphigus, etc.) are alternative diagnoses for which the topography of the lesions and the results of immunofluorescence are decisive . [29]
- In the sequellar stage of EPF, the differential diagnosis should be made with idiopathic eruptive macular pigmentation, which is an under-reported condition of unknown aetiology. Clinically composed of benign hyperpigmented macules, this condition is characterised histopathologically by dermal melanisation. It must be differentiated from lichen planus pigmentosa, erythema dyschromicum persans and mastocytosis pigmentosa .[30,31]

1.7.3. Aetiological diagnosis

The etiological diagnosis of toxidermia requires a drug causation approach. There are several methods, including that of *Bégaud*. This consists of using intrinsic and extrinsic criteria to determine drug liability. Several drugs can be attributed to EPF, including acetaminophen, NSAIDs and anti-infectious sulphonamides.

NB: any drug can cause toxidermia, and the list of compounds is not exhaustive.

Intrinsic accountability

Linked to the characteristics of the clinical picture :

- The appearance of the skin accident (semiological imputability)
- The chronology of the skin accident (chronological imputability)
- Delay between the introduction of the suspected drug and the onset of dermatitis,

- Progression after stopping the drug,
- Possibly the time between reintroduction and a new accident.
- Reintroduction may be involuntary; it may only be intentional in the case of benign toxidermia for which an essential drug is suspected.
- Chronological criteria

R+: positive rechallenge, R0: rechallenge not done, R-: negative rechallenge; C3: probable chronology, C2: plausible chronology, C1: doubtful chronology, C0: incompatible chronology.

Table II : semiological criteria of intrinsic imputability according to Bégaud in 1985

Semiological criteria	
Pharmacodynamic explanation (mechanism of action)	Evocative of the role of the drug or favouring factor
Contributing factors	Other situation
Possible differential diagnoses	No Yes
Complementary laboratory tests proving the drug cause	Positive Not done Negative

Extrinsic accountability

From the literature :

- Databases (paper, Internet) ;
- Specialist books ;
- Pharmaceutical laboratory ;
- Regional pharmacovigilance centres

Scores can be established, indicating the level of probability of responsibility of a given drug

TableII : Decision table combining chronological (C) and semiological (S) criteria in the French imputability method (Bégaud) updated in 2011

	TIME OF OCCURRENCE		
	Very suggestive	Compatible	Incompatible
Rechallenge	R (+) R (0) R (-)	R (+) R (0) R (-)	
EVOLUTION			
Suggestive	C3 C3 C1	C3 C2 C1	C0
Inconclusive	C3 C2 C1	C3 C1 C1	C0
Non-suggestive	C1 C1 C1	C1 C1 C0	C0

C3: Likely chronology
C2: Plausible chronology
C1 : Questionable chronology
C0: Incompatible chronology

SEMIOLOGY	Evocative of the role of the drug or factors Contributing situations		
SPECIFIC TEST		L(+) L(0) L(-)	L(+) L(0) L(-)
Non-medicinal causes	Absent Possible (or sought)	S3 S3 S1 S3 S2 S1	S3 S3 S1 S3 S1 S1

S3: Likely semiology
S2: Plausible semiology
S1: Questionable semiology

The results of the two previous decision tables are used as input for a third final table which gives the intrinsic imputability with 5 possible scores from 10 to 14.

TableIII : Decision table combining the chronological and semiological criteria in the French imputability method (Bégaud) updated in 2011

		SEMIOLOGY		
		S1	**S2**	**S3**
Timeline	**C0**	I0	I0	I0
	C1	I1	I1	I3
	C2	I1	I2	I3
	C3	I3	I3	I4

The answers to these 4 questions are used to calculate a semiological score from S1 to S3.

Finally, the calculation of intrinsic imputability **(I0**: excluded; **I1**: doubtful; **I2**: plausible; **I3**: probable; **I4**: very probable) is obtained by combining the chronological (C) and semiological (S) scores.

WHO method

Used by WHO National Collaborating Centres since 1987.

Advantage :

- Is internationally accepted
- Is easy to use

This method is largely based on 3 considerations:

- the chronological relationship between the administration of the medicinal product and the adverse event
- medical or pharmacological probability (signs and symptoms, laboratory tests, pathological data, mechanisms)
- presence or absence of other causes

Extrinsic accountability

The calculation of extrinsic imputability is relatively easy. It is based on bibliography (hence the B) and is rated in 4 groups from B0 to B3.

- B0: adverse reaction never reported ;
- B1: effect not published in standard treatises ;
- B2: rare effect, but published ;
- B3: effect known and well described (Vidal or treatises).

Intrinsic accountability

- calculating intrinsic imputability is a little more difficult.

  This calculation is based on the answers to 3 questions for the calculation of chronological imputability and 4 questions for semiological imputability.
- the 3 chronological questions are :

  1. Is the time between administration of the drug and the occurrence of the adverse event highly suggestive, compatible or incompatible?
  2. The evolution of the unexpected effect after stopping the drug: is it suggestive, inconclusive or not suggestive?
  3. Re-administration of the drug: is it positive, negative, not done or not assessable?

  The answers to these 3 questions are used to calculate a chronological score rated from 0 to 3.
- the 4 semiological questions are :

  1. Does the semiology itself indicate the role of the drug?
  2. Is there a highly favourable, well-validated factor (for toxidermia, the usual answer is no)?
  3. Is there another, non-drug explanation?
  4. Is a specific and reliable complementary test positive or negative?

1.8. Treatment

1.8.1. Curative treatment

1.8.1.1. Purpose

- Stop the suspect drug
- Relieving patients and preventing complications
- Issue a drug allergy card and a list of prohibited and authorised medicines

1.8.1.2. Resources

Fixed erythema pigmentosa, like all toxidermia, can be treated according to a single principle: avoidance of the imputed molecule and symptomatic treatment. The literature and reference books on the therapeutic management of EPF remain poor. he treatment of EPF must be based primarily on the identification and elimination of the molecule responsible for a given patient.

Specific treatment is based on cutaneous and/or mucosal symptoms: in the presence of bullous or erosive lesions, strong to very strong class dermocorticoids are recommended, depending on the intensity[32–35] .

1.8.2. Preventive treatment

1.8.2.1. Primary prevention

It consists of avoiding medicines that cause it.

1.8.2.2. Secondary prevention

Secondary prevention consists of avoiding complications (eczematisation, impetiginisation) once the disease has already occurred.

1.8.2.3 Tertiary prevention

This involves the creation of drug allergy cards or certificates listing the pharmacological class of the drug concerned and other similar drugs in the same family to be avoided. In this context, specify the molecules for which the patient is eligible.

2. STUDY FRAMEWORK AND METHODS

2.1. Background study

Our study took place in three dermatology and venereology centres:

2.1.1. University Dermatology and Venereology Clinic at the CNHU -HKM in Cotonou

The Dermatology and Venereology Department was created in June 1980. It was directed by **Professor Florencia do ANGO PADONOU** until September 2011 and then by the late **Professor Hubert YEDOMON** until January 2015. At present, it has been merged with the Dermatology Department of the Hôpital d'Instruction des Armées (HIA) and is under the direction of **Professor Félix ATADOKPEDE**. It changed its name in 2022 to become the Clinique Universitaire de Dermatologie-Vénérologie (CUDEV). It is staffed by a full professor of dermatology and venereology, who is head of department, an associate lecturer, a dermatologist, two state-qualified nurses, a secretary and an orderly. The clinic is open every working day from 7.30am to 5pm. It receives consultations by appointment and deals with all cases of dermatitis from different regions of the country and from other departments of the CNHU/HKM. In addition to dermatological consultations, local treatments are administered and dermatological surgery is performed. Patients are hospitalised in other departments, as the department does not yet have an inpatient ward. As part of its clinical and teaching activities, the department provides training for doctors specialising in dermatology and venereology. It also welcomes Master 1 general medicine and INMES students.

2.1.2. Dermatology Department of the Buruli Ulcer Screening and Treatment Centre in Allada

The Buruli Ulcer Screening and Treatment Centre in Allada is located in the Atlantic department. The centre was inaugurated on 8 July 2002. It is the creation of the Fondation Follereau Luxembourg. It contains several hospital wards with a capacity of 80 beds, several consultation offices, a large meeting room, a radiology and medical imaging department, an operating theatre with two operating theatres, a recovery and sterilisation room, a laboratory, two large dressing rooms, an orthopaedic equipment room, an administrative building and a kitchen. Since 2023, it has been run by a Dermatology-Venerology department headed by an Associate Professor and assisted by three state-qualified nurses and doctors specialising in Dermatology. The department operates 24 hours a day, with consultations from 8am to 6pm.

2.1.3. Centre Médical la Providence, Cotonou

This is a private dermatology and venereology practice located in the Houéyiho district of Cotonou. It is run by a dermatology and venereology doctor, assisted by two nurses, two beauticians and a secretary. The practice's main activities include dermatology and venereology consultations, as well as specialised dermatology, allergology and surgery.

It is open Monday to Friday from 8.00 am to 6.00 pm and Saturday from 8.00 am to 1.00 pm.

2.2 Study methods

2.2.1. Type of study

This was a cross-sectional study with retrospective and prospective multicentre data collection.

2.2.2. Study period

The study covered an eleven (11) year period from January 2013 to November 2024. Data were collected for the retrospective part from 08 August 2024 to 15 September 2024 and for the prospective part from 16 September to 30 November 202 4.

NB: The data were collected as follows:

- CUDEV since January 2013.
- CMP since June 2015.

- CDTUB - Allada since November 2023.

2.2.3. Population studied

The study population consisted of patients consulting the CUDEV, the CDTUB and the CMP for EPF during the study period.

2.2.4. Selection criteria

2.2.4.1. Inclusion criteria

Any patient of any sex or age seen in the period from January 2013 to November 2024 who meets the EPF's clinical criteria.

2.2.4.2. Non-inclusion criteria

All incomplete files, with a diagnosis of toxidermia other than EPF.

2.2.5. Sampling

This was a non-probability sample with exhaustive identification of all cases of EPF.

2.2.6. Study variables

2.2.6.1. Dependent variable

The only dependent variable in our study is the diagnosis of EPF.

2.2.6.2. Independent variables

- **Socio-demographic variables**
    - **Age**: the time elapsed between a person's birth and a given date; a point in life corresponding to this time (in years).
    - **Sex**: the physical characteristics that distinguish males from females and males from females.
    - **Ethnic group**: a group of people who share a number of civilisational characteristics, particularly culture and language.

- **Profession**: state, trade, job from which one derives one's means of existence and subsistence.
- **Residence**: the place where you usually live.

- **Variables linked to habits**
  - Self-medication
  - Sexual habits: number of partners, type of sex, whether or not condoms are used, etc.
  - Cosmetic habits (depigmentation)
  - Eating habits: type of food eaten by patients
- **Clinical variables**
  - Date of onset of illness (in days)
  - Year of consultation: 2013 to 2024
  - Reason for consultation: fluid lesions, black spots, localised pruritus, localised pain.
  - Sites of injury : head, neck, thoracic region, lumbar region, sacral region, abdominal region, thoracic limbs, pelvic limbs, OGE, damage to mucous membranes, multiple sites
  - Personal and family history
  - Number of lesions: single, 2 to 5, more than 5
  - Evolution :
    - favourable if the drug involved is stopped and dermocorticoids are applied. Healing of the lesions occurred at the cost of residual pigmentation.
    - unfavourable if, after stopping the drug, complications due to the disease persist, such as synechia of the mucous membranes or semi-mucous membranes, extension of lesions and impetiginisation.
  - Diagnosis chosen/clinical forms of EPF (bullous EPF, generalized EPF, non-pigmented EPF, common form of EPF)

- Complications: impetiginisation, eczematisation, ulceration, hyperpigmented sequelae, hypopigmentation, death
- Previous treatment and paraclinical investigations carried out

2.2.7. Data collection

2.2.7.1. Source

Data were collected from various registers and patient files. Some paraclinical investigations were carried out, especially in subjects with several drugs involved.

2.2.7.2. Tools

The main data collection tool was the pre-established, digitised survey form.

2.2.7.3. Collection technique

This involved a retrospective review of patient records, taking data directly from registers and patients' physical and electronic files.

2.2.7.4. Survey team

It was made up of a doctor in his fourth year of specialising in dermatology and venereology, a general practitioner and a sixth-year medical student. The survey team was trained in the research protocol.

2.2.7.5. Conduct of the survey

Patients were included according to their years of consultation, starting in January 2013 and ending in November 2024, taking into account our inclusion criteria. Each file included was given a number in our manual data collection form. After checking and filling in the required information, the data was entered into the database, which was updated daily via smartphones.

2.2.8. Data processing and analysis

At the end of data collection, the forms were manually analysed to check that they were complete and that the data had been filled in consistently. The data was then entered into the Kobocollect software.

The data were analysed using *Jamovi* software. Text processing and the creation of tables and graphs were carried out using Microsoft Word and Excel version 2013.

2.2.9. Ethical and deontological considerations

This work was carried out in accordance with current ethical and deontological standards. The data were collected, entered and analysed with the strictest anonymity. Patients were identified by a number assigned to them once their file had been accepted for the study.

3. RESULTS

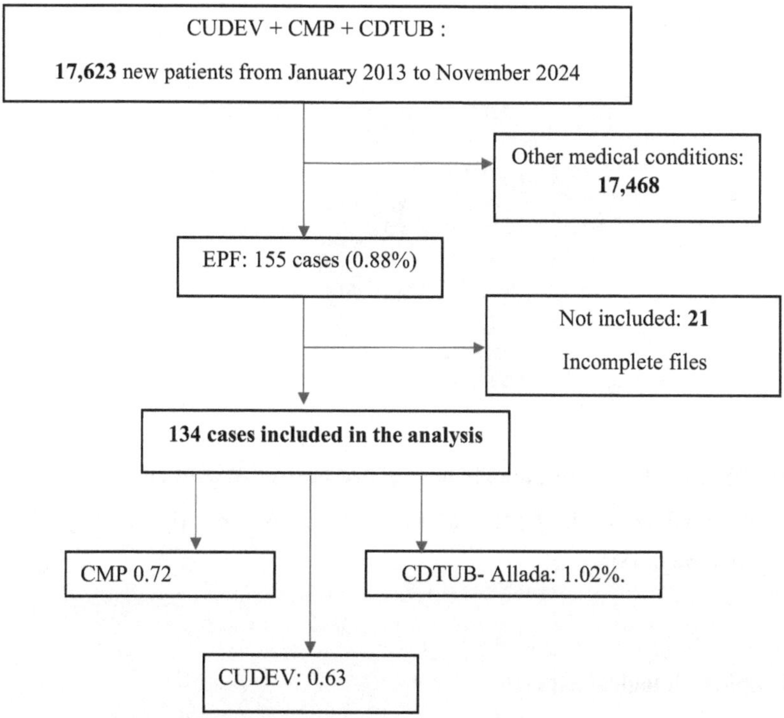

Figure8 : flow chart of the study

3.1. Prevalence overall and by centre

The three centres (CNHU-HKM, CMP and CDTUB-Allada) received a total of 17,623 new patients, including 155 with EPF, giving an overall hospital incidence rate of 0.88%.

For the retrospective part, a total of 121 cases out of 134, i.e. 90.29%, and a total of 13 cases out of 134, i.e. 9.7%, for the prospective part.

3.2 Care centre

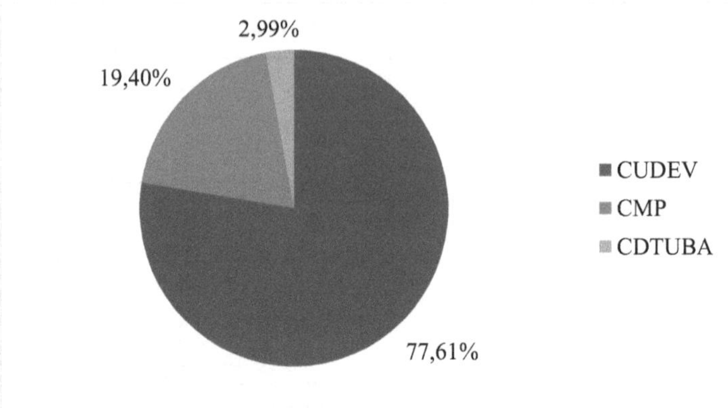

Figure9 : distribution of patients having had an EPF according to the centre of care at the CUDEV, the CMP and the CDTUB- Allada from January 2013 to November 2024 (N= 134) .

3.3. Epidemiological aspects

3.3.1. Year

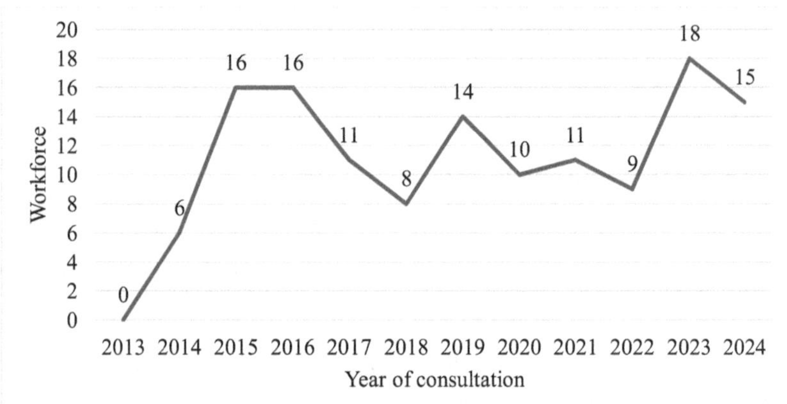

Figure10 : distribution of patients who had an EPF according to the year of consultation at the CUDEV, the CMP and the CDTUB- Allada from January 2013 to November 2024 (N= 134) .

3.3.2. Age

The mean age of the patients was 35.87 ± 20.27 years, with extremes of 1 year and 89 years .

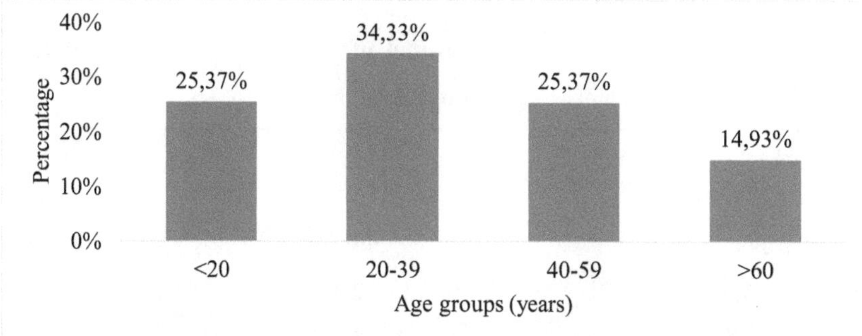

Figure11 : distribution of patients having had an EPF according to age at the CUDEV, the CMP and the CDTUB- Allada from January 2013 to November 2024 (N= 134)

3.3.3. Sex

Of the 134 subjects, 76 (56.72%) were male, with an M/F sex ratio of 1.31.

3.3.4. Profession

TableIV : distribution of patients having had an EPF according to profession at the CUDEV, the CMP and the CDTUB- Allada from January 2013 to November 2024 (N= 134)

	Number of employees (n)	Proportion
Pupil/Student	34	25,37
Civil servant	34	25,37
Not specified	27	20,15
Trade	24	17,91
Unemployed	15	11,19
Total	**134**	**100,0**

3.3.5. Source

Table VV : distribution of patients having had an EPF according to department of origin at the CUDEV, the CMP and the CDTUB- Allada from January 2013 to November 2024 (N= 134)

	Number of employees (n)	Proportion
Coastal / Atlantic	121	90,30
Ouémé / Plateau	5	3,73
Zou / Hills	3	2,24
Atacora / Donga	2	1,49
Mono / Couffo	2	1,49
Alibori / Borgou	1	0, 75
Total	**134**	**100,0**

3.3.6. Place of residence

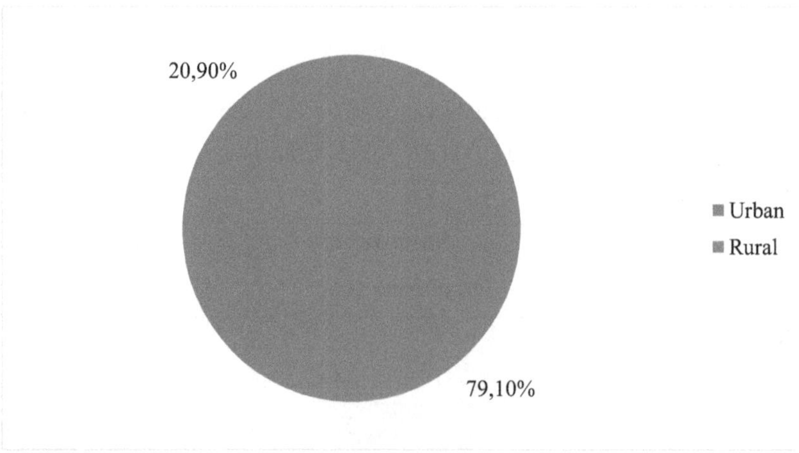

Figure12 : distribution of patients having had an EPF according to place of residence at the CUDEV, at the CMP and at the CDTUB- Allada from January 2013 to November 2024 (N= 134)

3.4. Clinical aspects

3.4.1. Reason for consultation

TableVI : distribution of patients having had an EPF according to the reason for consultation at the CUDEV, the CMP and the CDTUB- Allada from January 2013 to November 2024 (N= 134)

	Number of employees (n)	Proportion
Black spots	78	58,21
Liquid lesions	20	14,92
Localised pruritus	22	16,42
Localised pain	14	10,44

3.4.2. Personal atopy

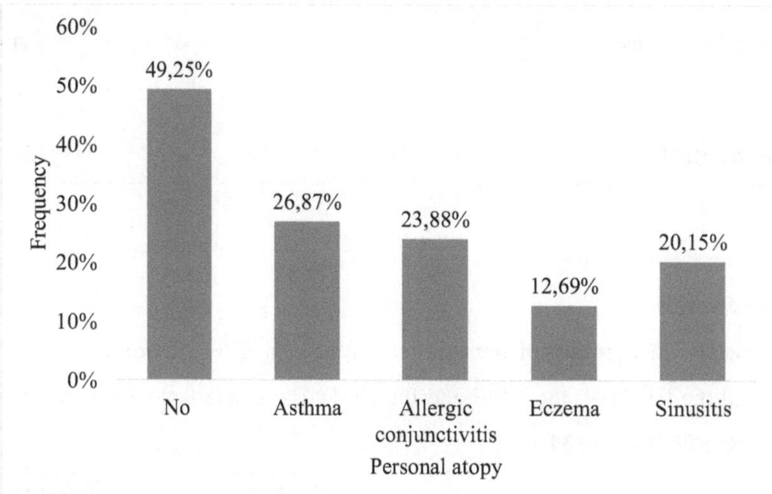

Figure13 : Distribution of patients having had an EPF according to the existence of atopic manifestations at the CUDEV, the CMP and the CDTUB- Allada from January 2013 to November 2024 (N=134)

3.4.3. Medical history

TableVII : distribution of patients having had an EPF according to comorbidities at the CUDEV, the CMP and the CDTUB- Allada from January 2013 to November 2024 (N= 134)

	Number of employees (n)	**Proportion**
Systemic lupus erythematosus	5	3,73
HTA	16	11,94
Diabetes	12	8,96
HIV infection	5	3,73
Hepatopathy	6	4,48
Nephropathies	11	8,21
Rheumatoid arthritis	6	4,48
Sickle cell disease	6	4,48
Atopy	28	20,89
Not specified	39	29,12

3.4.4 Lifestyle

TableVIII : distribution of patients having had an EPF according to personal habits at the CUDEV, the CMP and the CDTUB- Allada from January 2013 to November 2024 (N= 134)

	Number of employees (n)	**Proportion**

Alcoholism	18	13,43
Drug addiction	3	2,24
Not specified	83	61,94

3.4.5. Episode

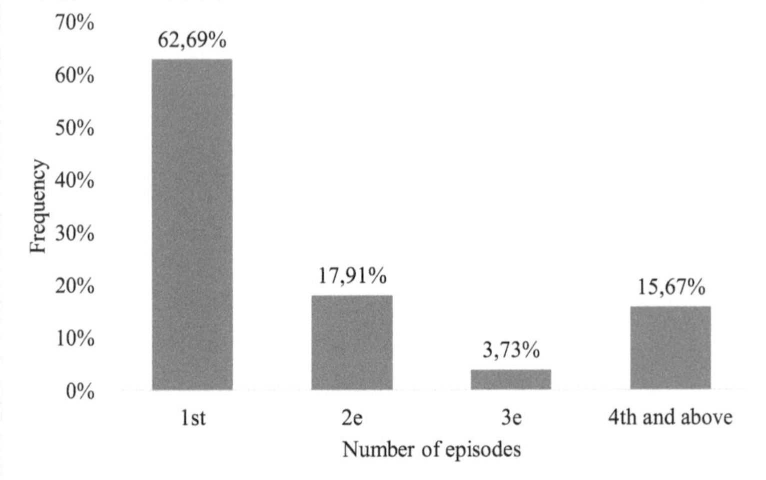

Figure14 : distribution of patients who had an EPF according to the number of episodes at the CUDEV , the CMP and the CDTUB- Allada from January 2013 to November 2024 (N=134)

3.4.6. Time to onset

TableIX : distribution of patients having had an EPF according to the usual waiting time at the CUDEV, CMP and CDTUB- Allada from January 2013 to November 2024 (N=134)

	Number of employees (n)	Proportion
Less than 24 hours	22	16,42
24H - 48H	30	22,39
More than 48 hours	82	61,19
Total	**134**	**100,0**

3.4.7. Clinical forms

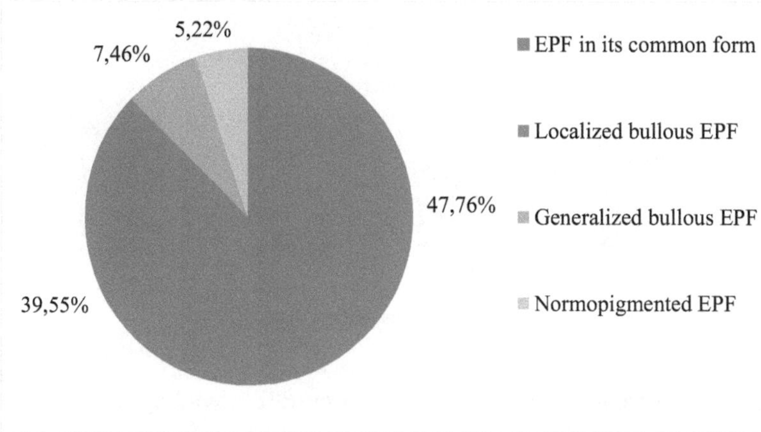

Figure15 : distribution of patients with EPF according to clinical form .

3.4.8. Factors involved

Table XX : distribution of patients with an EPF according to the drug or food in question at CUDEV, CMP and CDTUB- Allada from January 2013 to November 2024 (N=134)

	Number of employees (n)	Proportion
Medicines		
Paracetamol	49	36,56
CTA	31	23,13
Cotrimoxazole	29	21, 64
Food in question		
Moringa leaf	7	5,22
Licorice	3	2,24
Ginger	2	1,49
Causes not found	13	9,70

3.4.9. Consultation time after appearance of lesion

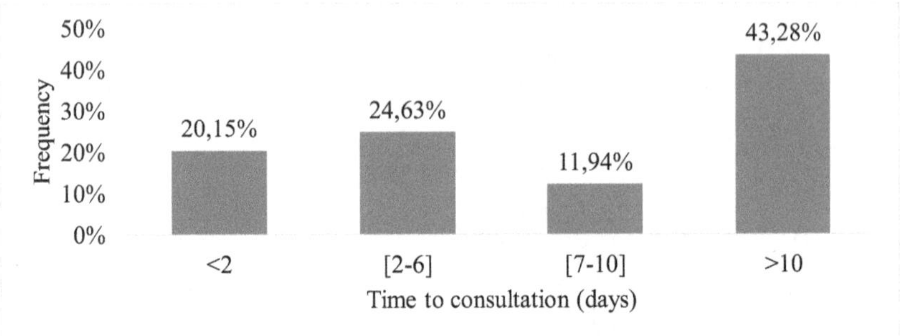

Figure16 : distribution of patients having had an EPF according to the delay before consultation at the CUDEV, the CMP and the CDTUB- Allada from January 2013 to November 2024 (N=134)

3.4.10. Therapeutic itinerary

TableXI : distribution of patients having had an EPF according to itinerary

	Number of employees (n)	Proportion
Home - self-medication - hospital		59,70
Home - Hospital	53	39,55
Home - traditional practitioner - hospital	1	0,75
Total	**134**	**100,0**

3.4.11. Immediate behaviour

TableXII I: distribution of patients having had an EPF according to the immediate attitude adopted after the occurrence of lesions at the CUDEV, CMP and CDTUB-Allada from January 2013 to November 2024 (N=177)

	Number of employees (n)	Proportion
Call the doctor	43	32,09
Replaced by another drug	6	4,48
Stopping the drug	36	26,87
Continuation of treatment	84	62,69
No action	8	5,97

3.4.12. Conditions requiring medication

Table XIIIXIII : distribution of patients having had an EPF according to the illness causing the medication) at the CUDEV, CMP and CDTUB- Allada from January 2013 to November 2024 (N=134)

	Number of employees (n)	Proportion
No disease reported	**101**	**75,37**
Yes	**33**	**24,63**
Malaria	12	8,96
Cough	4	2,99
Joint pain	2	1,49
Flu	1	0,75
Breast cancer	1	0,75
Hypertension	1	0,75
Sickle cell vaso-occlusive crisis	1	0,75
Fever of unspecified aetiology	1	0,75
Diarrhoea	1	0,75
HTA	1	0,75
Sepsis	1	0,75
Arthralgia	1	0,75

Manic episodes	1	0,75
HIV	1	0,75
Toxoplasmosis in HIV	1	0,75
Enteritis	1	0,75
Retromalleolar abscess	1	0,75
Diaper rash	1	0,75

3.4.13. Location of lesions

Table XIVXIV : distribution of patients having had an EPF according to the site of the lesions at the CUDEV, the CMP and the CDTUB- Allada from January 2013 to November 2024 (N=13 4)

	Number of employees (n)	**Proportion**
Head	26	19,40
Neck	10	7,46
Thoracic region	35	26,12
Sacred region	12	8,96
Pelvic limb	49	36,57
General	7	5,22
Thoracic limb	39	29,10
EMB	28	20,90
Abdominal region	20	14,93
Lumbar region	7	5,22
Multiple seating	57	42,54
Mucosal damage	14	10 ,44

3.4.14. Elementary injuries

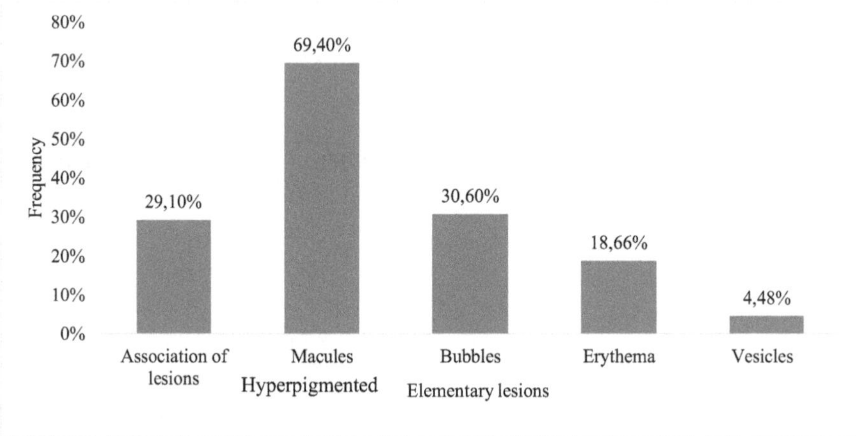

Figure17 : distribution of patients having had an EPF according to elementary lesions at the CUDEV, the CMP and the CDTUB- Allada from January 2013 to November 2024 (N=134) .

3.4.15. Number of lesions on the body

TableXV : distribution of patients having had an EPF according to the number of lesions at the CUDEV, the CMP and the CDTUB- Allada from January 2013 to November 2024 (N=134)

	Number of employees (n)	Proportion
Not specified	8	5,97
1-2	37	27,61
3-4	25	18,66
5-6	18	13,43
7-8	11	8,21
9-10	10	7,46
>11	25	18,66

Total	**134**	**100,0**

3.4.16. Body surface area affected

TableXVI : distribution of patients who had an EPF according to the skin surface affected at the CUDEV, the CMP and the CDTUB- Allada from January 2013 to November 2024 (N=134) .

	Number of employees (n)	Proportion
Not specified	24	17,91
10% SCA	78	58,21
SCA 10% - 20% DISCOUNT	19	14,18
ACS > 30% OF THE TIME	13	9,70
Total	**134**	**100,0**

3.4.17. Paraclinical work-up

TableXVII : distribution of patients having had an EPF according to the paraclinical assessment at the CUDEV, the CMP and the CDTUB- Allada from January 2013 to November 2024 (N=134) .

	Number of employees (n)	Proportion
HIV serology (N=10)		
HIV positive	9	9/10
Fasting blood glucose (N=10)		
Diabetes	4	4/10
CBC (N=20)		
Microcytic anaemia	2	2/20
Hyperleukocytosis	3	3/20
Lymphopenia	1	1/20
Neutropenia	4	4/20
Normal	10	10/20

Hepatitis B serology (N=5)		
Viral hepatitis B	1	1/4
Patch test (N=7)		
Patch test	5	5/7
Skin biopsy (N=1)		
Histopathology in favour	1	1/1
Negative	-	0/1

3.4.18. Drug imputability using the Bégaud method et al

Of the 134 cases, 82.17% were very likely, 5.97% likely and 11.86% unspecified.

3.5. Therapeutic aspects

3.5.1. Drug allergy certificate

TableXVIII : distribution of patients having had an EPF according to the existence of the eviction certificate at the CUDEV, the CMP and the CDTUB-Allada from January 2013 to November 2024 (N=134)

	Number of employees (n)	Proportion
Elaborated	66	49,25
Not seen	66	49,25
Viewed at	2	1,49
Total	**134**	**100,0**

3.5.2. Treatment

TableXIX : distribution of patients having had an EPF according to drug treatments at the CUDEV, the CMP and the CDTUB- Allada from January 2013 to November 2024 (N=134)

	Number of employees (n)	Proportion
Emollients	94	70,15
Antiseptics	66	49,25
Antihistamines	42	31,34
Dermocorticoids	25	18,66
Antibiotics	18	13,43
Analgesics	9	6,72

3.6. Prognostic aspects

3.6.1. Evolutionary mode

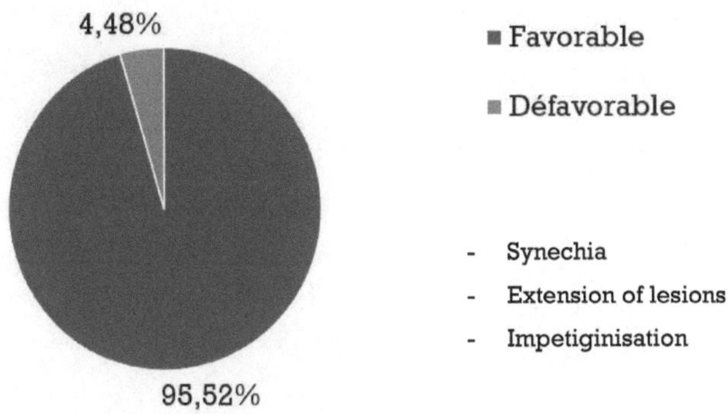

Figure18 : distribution of patients having had an EPF according to progress at the CUDEV, the CMP and the CDTUB- Allada from January 2013 to November 2024 (N=134)

3.6.2. Complications

TableXX : distribution of patients having had an EPF according to complications at the CUDEV, the CMP and the CDTUB- Allada from January 2013 to November 2024 (N=134)

	Number of employees (n)	**Proportion**
Ulceration or erosions	43	32 ,08
Impetiginisation	36	26, 86
Eczema	28	20,89
Deaths	3	2, 23
Not specified	24	18, 02

3.6.3. Appointments

Of the 134 cases, 53.73% kept their appointments and 46.27% were lost to follow-up.

4. DISCUSSION

We will approach this chapter as follows:

- Achieving the study objectives
- Validity and quality of results
- Commentary, interpretation and comparison of results

4.1. Achieving objectives

At the end of our study, we can consider that the objectives set have been achieved.

We were able to :

- To determine the incidence of erythema pigmentum fixans in hospitals in Cotonou and Allada and at the CMP.
- To describe the epidemiological, clinical and therapeutic features of erythema pigmentum fixans at the CUDEV, the CMP and the CDTUB in Allada
- Identifying the drugs responsible for EPF

4.2. Validity and quality of results

The questionnaire was designed to determine the incidence of EPF in three coastal and Atlantic hospitals, and all the study investigators were duly trained in the methodology. The data were collected, recorded and stored in strict compliance with the rules of medical ethics and deontology. However, a number of biases need to be taken into account when interpreting our results, in particular the retrospective nature of the study. Our study was confronted with certain limitations linked to its retrospective nature, namely :

- missing data,
- uncertainty about the data in the files,
- Difficulty in carrying out an aetiological investigation (patch tests and drug imputability not carried out)

Despite these limitations, our study is interesting because it provided data on the epidemiological, clinical and therapeutic features of EPF in three health centres in Cotonou and Allada.

4.3. Comparison of results with those of other authors

- **Incidence**

The incidence of EPF was 0.88% in our study. Yu -Ju - Chu in 2022 in Taiwan found a prevalence of 14-22% of toxidermia in the paediatric population[36] . This difference with us could be explained by the fact that our study populations are different. Our population was made up of new patients, but his was made up of children only.

4.3.1. Socio-demographic factors associated with EPF

- **Age**

The mean age of our patients was 35.87 ± 20.27 years. This result is similar to that of Ravinder in India in 2015, who found the age to be 37.5 ± 11.26 years, but different from that of Koutou in Cameroon in 2017 (41.07 ± 11.2) 6 years. This difference in ages is explained by the larger sample size for our study and that of Ravinder, but smaller for Kouotou et al. and also our study populations are different, in our study and that of Ravinder, it consisted of new patients, but Kouotou had worked on people living with HIV.

- **Profession**

Our study showed that schoolchildren were the most affected, with 25.37%. This result is similar to that found by **Atadokpèdé et al**. *in* Benin in 2009[11] . Traders are much more exposed to the risk factor of self-medication. Traders are very preoccupied with their business and prefer to treat their ailments symptomatically rather than consulting a doctor, which explains their high exposure to self-medication[37] .

- **History**

The majority of patients in our study had an atopic manifestation, either asthma, sinusitis, allergic conjunctivitis or simply atopic dermatitis (constitutional eczema). The association of this toxidermia with atopic dermatitis has not yet been clearly elucidated in the literature. Some authors, such as **Ordoqui et al** in 1995 in France[38] and **Haifa Ben et al.** in 2019 in Tunisia[39] , speak of cross-effects.

4.3.2. Clinical aspects

- **Reason for consultation**

More than half of the patients in our study consulted for black spots (58.21%). This result is different from that of **Garcia et al** in 2017 in Spain and **Monelli et al** in 2019 in Italy who found in their series liquid lesions such as bullae as reasons for consultation. This could be explained by the different clinical forms in our studies. In our series, the common form was more represented than the generalised bullous and localised bullous forms in the studies by **Garcia** and Monelli respectively.

- **Itinerary**

The route taken by the majority of patients in our series was home - self-medication - hospital. This result differs from that of **Slim et al** in Tunisia, where in 2021 patients had a home-hospital itinerary. This difference can be explained by the accessibility to care due to a higher universal health coverage in Tunisia to 83% of the population in 2022 . [40]

- **Appearance of the hyperpigmented macule**

EPF is one of the toxidermias with the characteristic of leaving sequelae that allow a retrospective diagnosis. The appearance of lesions in the same places allows this retrospection and makes the diagnosis of EPF. [41] . Our results are in the same vein, the diagnosis of EPF in our patients was also made thanks to the sequellar lesions which also constituted their reason for consultation as described in 2019 by **Singh Vikramjeet et al** in India and **L. Sanchez et al** in 2013 in Spain . [42,43]

- **Time to onset of lesions**

Seventy-one point nine percent of our patients noticed their lesion after taking the drug for 4 days or more. This result differs from the majority of studies in the literature. This difference could be explained by three reasons: in our series, we have a predominantly male sex ratio when we know that men do not consult too much in our context, but also the practice of self-medication which lengthens the consultation time and thirdly the difference in phenotypes of our patients who were all of phototype VI contrary to those of **Ratinder et al** in India in 2018 and **Januat et al** in Bangladesh in 2023.

- **Number of lesions**

Concerning the number of lesions in our patients, 61% had less than two lesions and 5.97% had lesions with an unspecified number. This result is similar to that of **Kououtou E et al** in 2017 in Cameroon [41], who found 52.2% of patients with more than 3 lesions. This difference could be explained by the fact that our study populations all came mainly from urban areas and they had all consulted the hospital early. Also, the majority of patients in both studies were experiencing their first episodes.

- **Evolution**

The outcome was favourable in 95.52% of cases. This result is similar to that of **Joachim et al** in 2017 in France [47]. This similarity can be explained by the fact that the course of EPF is generally benign, becoming unfavourable in the presence of synechiae, extension of lesions and impetiginisation.

- **Clinical forms**

In our series, the common form of EPF was 47.76%. This result is similar to that of **Atadokpèdé et al** in 2009 in Benin, **Saka et al** in 2012 in Togo and **Koutou et al** in 2017 in Cameroon. This similarity could be explained by the identity of the phototype of our patients but also by the fact that in all these studies, the common form of EPF predominated. On the other hand, few studies mentioned the normopigmented form, as was the case in our study. This rarity could be explained by the diagnostic difficulty of this form of EPF.

4.3.3. Drug involved

Paracetamol was the most frequently incriminated drug at 36.56%.

This result differs from that of **Atadokpèdé et al** in 2009 in Benin and **Saka et al** in 2012 in Togo, who all found anti-infectious sulphonamides followed by NSAIDs. Paracetamol as the primary cause of EPF in Benin suggests several hypotheses: a poorly conducted aetiological investigation and/or a change in the epidemiology of toxidermia in Benin.

4.3.4. Paraclinical aspects

The diagnosis of EPF, like that of other toxidermias, is primarily clinical. Certain tests may be carried out to provide guidance and, above all, to diagnose comorbidities. In our study, we did some of these:

Nine out of 134 patients in our series had positive HIV retroviral serology. This result differs from that of **Kououtou E et al** in 2017 who found 3 out of 41 or 1.4%[44] and **Ravinder Kaur** in 2016 in the United Kingdom [56] who found 0.7%[45] . **Sharon L in** 2013 in Ireland had a proportion of 1.5%[63] . This difference could be explained by the different methodology of each of these studies and the duration of the work, but above all by the different epidemiology of HIV in these countries. EPF, like all toxidermia, is one of the dermatological manifestations leading to the discovery of HIV infection. This is why HIV serology should be sought in all cases of toxidermia in general, and EPF in particular . [23]

- **Patch tests**

Three point seven three percent of the patients in our study had a positive patch test. This result is in line with the literature, which states that the only test that can reveal the responsibility of a drug is the patch test (patch test, prick test and intradermal reaction)[23,47,48] . In our context, only the patch test was used in 3.73% of cases, which shows that we still have a long way to go, but also that the absence of these tests in our environments encourages a clinical approach to the diagnosis of this toxidermia . [49]

- **Histopathology**

Skin biopsy and histopathological examination were performed in 0.75% of patients in our series. As histopathology is an essential examination for this condition, the few times it was performed in our study, it was often in the non-pigmented form of EPF, which posed the problem of differential diagnosis. Our results are in line with the numerous data in the literature on this subject [36,67]

4.3.5. Therapeutic aspects

In our 42 patients were treated with antihistamines, 25 with dermocorticoids and 25 with topical antiseptics and 9 were treated with an analgesic. These results are in line with those of **Saka et al** in 2012 in Togo[37] and **Atadokpèdé et al** in 2009 in Benin[11] . This similarity could be explained by the fact that these two studies were all carried out in specialist dermatology centres.

CONCLUSION AND SUGGESTIONS

CONCLUSION

The study showed that the hospital prevalence of EPF was low. The extreme ages were 1 year and 89 years. The most common age group was 20 to 39. High blood pressure was the most common comorbidity. The majority of patients were first-time sufferers. The time to onset of lesions was between 24 and 48 hours in the majority of patients. Paracetamol was the main chemical agent involved. Moringa leaves and ginger were the main food sources. The route taken by the majority of patients was home - self-medication - hospital. Most stopped taking the medication as soon as the symptoms appeared. The hyperpigmented macule was the most common elementary lesion. A drug allergy certificate was drawn up for the majority of patients. Ulceration or erosion was the most common complication.

SUGGESTIONS

At the end of our work, our suggestions are as follows:

- **To the public**
    - Avoid self-medication
    - Any sudden appearance of hyperpigmented macules should be reported as soon as possible.
    - Always be able to record in a personal diary any medication taken and its timing.

- **For nurses, general practitioners and specialists other than dermatologists**
    - Updating theoretical knowledge and learning more about the various diagnostic approaches to EPF, as well as unusual clinical forms.
    - Refer cases to specialist services as soon as possible if in doubt.

- **To Pharmacists**
    - Always be able to ask patients for drug allergy certificates before selling them a drug, and refer them to a doctor for proper management, because the same causes produce the same effects.
    - Discourage the practice of buying medicines without a prescription signed by a doctor.

- **For specialists in Dermatology-Venerology**

  Promote ongoing training with doctors from other specialities to enable them to update their theoretical knowledge.
- **To the political and administrative authorities**

  Ensure compliance with the regulations governing the sale of medicines, by requiring pharmacies to provide allergy certificates where they exist, and also to ensure that medicines are only sold on prescriptions duly signed by a doctor on the medical register.

REFERENCES

1. Anderson HJ, Lee JB. A Review of Fixed Drug Eruption with a Special Focus on Generalized Bullous Fixed Drug Eruption. Med Kaunas Lith. 1 Sep 2021;57(9):925.

2. Özkaya E. Fixed drug eruption: state of the art. JDDG J Dtsch Dermatol Ges. March 2008 ;6(3):181-8.

3. Orchard DC, Varigos GA. Fixed drug eruption to tartrazine. Australas J Dermatol. 1997 ;38(4) :212-4.

4. Mahboob A, Haroon TS. Drugs causing fixed eruptions: a study of 450 cases. Int J Dermatol. Nov 1998 ;37(11) :833-8.

5. Yoboué P, Sangare A, Kaloga M, Kouadio A, Djedje MA. Epidemiologic and etiologic features of pigmentation disorders observed during consultation at the Dermatology Center of Abidjan, Ivory Coast. Int J Dermatol. oct 2005 ;44 Suppl 1 :33-4.

6. Alvarez VJ, Picón JE, Morales AR, Goncalves ET, Luna JR. [Fixed pigmented erythema related to the oral administration of carbamazepine: report of one case]. Invest Clin. March 2006;47(1):65-9.

7. Ohira A, Yamaguchi S, Miyagi T, Yamamoto YI, Yamada S, Shiohira H, et al. Fixed eruption due to quinine in tonic water: a case report with high-performance liquid chromatography and ultraviolet A analyses. J Dermatol. August 2013 ;40(8):629-31.

8. Taghy A, Zoobo T, Ismaili N, Senouci K, Hassam B. [Suspicion of food contaminants in the occurrence of a fixed drug eruption in a child]. Presse Medicale Paris Fr 1983. Mars 2015 ;44(3):365-7.

9. Valeyrie-Allanore L, Lebrun-Vignes B, Bensaid B, Sassolas B, Barbaub A. Erythema pigmentosum fixans: epidemiology, pathophysiology, clinic, differential diagnosis and management. Ann Dermatol Vénéréologie. 1 Nov 2015;142(11):701-6.

10. Zaouak A, Ben Salem F, Ben Jannet S, Hammami H, Fenniche S. Bullous fixed drug eruption : A potential diagnostic pitfall : a study of 18 cases. Therapies. 1 Oct 2019 ;74(5) :527-30.

11. Atadokpédé AF, Adégbidi H, Yédomon HG, Koudoukpo C, Agbessi N, Gnossike J, et al. Fixed erythema pigmentosum in Cotonou, Benin, from 1998 to 2008. Ann Dermatol Vénéréologie. 1 Apr 2011 ;138(4) :320-2.

12. Gupta A, Arora P, Malhotra P, Sardana K. Pheniramine maleate: an apparently safe drug causing bullous fixed drug eruption. Dermatol Online J. August 23, 2018 ;24(6):13030/qt1vc6p92x.

13. Assouère MN, Mazereeuw-Hautier J, Bonafé JL [Cutaneous drug eruption with two antihistaminic drugs of a same chemical family: cetirizine and hydroxyzine]. Ann Dermatol Venereol. Nov 2002 ;129(11) :1295-8.

14. Cravo M, Gonçalo M, Figueiredo A. Fixed drug eruption to cetirizine with positive lesional patch tests to the three piperazine derivatives. Int J Dermatol. Jul 2007 ;46(7):760-2.

15. Bhari N, Mahajan R, Singh S, Sharma VK. Fixed drug eruption due to three antihistamines of a same chemical family: Cetirizine, levocetirizine, and hydroxyzine. Dermatol Ther. March 2017;30(2).

16. Barbaud A. Allergological investigations in fixed erythema pigmentosum. Method recommended by the FISARD group of the SFD. Ann Dermatol Vénéréologie. 1 March 2018;145(3):210-3.

17. Pellicano R, Ciavarella G, Lomuto M, Di Giorgio G. Genetic susceptibility to fixed drug eruption: Evidence for a link with HLA-B22. J Am Acad Dermatol. 1 Jan 1994;30(1):52-4.

18. Khalili N. The Immunogenetics of Cutaneous Drug Reactions. Adv Exp Med Biol. 2022 ;1367:411-31.

19. Mitre V, Applebaum DS, Albahrani Y, Hsu S. Generalized bullous fixed drug eruption mimicking toxic epidermal necrolysis: a case report and literature review. Dermatol Online J. 15 Jul 2017 ;23(7):13030/qt25v009gs.

20. Bansal A, Kumari R, Ramam M. Fixed drug eruption due to cross reaction between two azoles used for different indications. Indian J Dermatol Venereol Leprol. 2008 ;74(1) :81.

21. Vocanson M, Tauber M, Villani AP, Nicolas JF. Pathophysiology of toxidermia. Lyell syndrome, a massive clonal expansion of polycytotoxic CD8+ T lymphocytes. Bull Académie Nat Médecine. 1 August 2023;207(7):910-6.

22. Bataille M, Vonarx M, Vermersch-Langlin A. Illustration of diagnostic and prognostic difficulties during the early stages of generalized bullous fixed drug eruptions. Eur J Dermatol. 1 Jan 2017 ;27(1) :86-8.

23. Braesch C, Gaudin O, Lebrun-Vignes B, Bernigaud C, Hua C, Ortonne N, et al. Recurrence of generalized erythema pigmentosum bullosa in the elderly: an example of a serious preventable medication error. Ann Dermatol Vénéréologie. 1 Dec 2020;147(12, Supplement): A163.

24. Chaabani M, Ben Salem F, Zaouak A, Ben Jannet S, Hammami H, Fenniche S. Genital involvement in bullous fixed erythema pigmentosum. Ann Dermatol Vénéréologie. May 1, 2018;145(4, Supplement): A55.

25. Tanabe K, Tsuboi H, Maejima H, Arai S, Katsuoka K. Non-pigmented fixed drug eruption induced by eprazinone hydrochloride. Dermatol Online J. 1 Dec 2005;11(3) :25.

26. Welfringer-Morin A, Bellon N, Milpied B, Bernier C. Toxidermia in children. Ann Dermatol Vénéréologie - FMC. 1 Nov 2022;2(8):616-24.

27. Sachdeva RK, Sharma A, De D, Malhi J, Rewari BB, Singh S, et al. Lamivudine-Induced Skin Rash Remains an Underdiagnosed Entity in HIV: A Case Series from a Single Center. J Int Assoc Provid AIDS Care. 2016;15(2):153-8.

28. Lebrun-Vignes B, Valeyrie-Allanore L. Toxidermia. Rev Médecine Interne. 1 Apr 2015 ;36(4):256-70.

29. Özkaya-Bayazit E. Specific site involvement in fixed drug eruption. J Am Acad Dermatol. 1 Dec 2003 ;49(6):1003-7.

30. Grover S, Basu A. Idiopathic eruptive macular pigmentation: report on two cases. Indian J Dermatol. 2010;55(3):277-8.

31. Jang KA, Choi JH, Sung KS, Moon KC, Koh JK. Idiopathic eruptive macular pigmentation: report of 10 cases. J Am Acad Dermatol. Feb 2001 ;44(2 Suppl) :351-3.

32. Ben Saad R, Souissi A, Karray M, Derbel F, Jellouli A, Dougui H. P 31: Erythema pigmentum fixata: a series of 10 cases. Ann Dermatol Venereologie. Apr 1, 2016;143(4, Supplement 1):S46.

33. Patel S, John AM, Handler MZ, Schwartz RA. Fixed Drug Eruptions: An Update, Emphasizing the Potentially Lethal Generalized Bullous Fixed Drug Eruption. Am J Clin Dermatol. June 2020;21(3):393-9.

34. Tripathy R, Pattnaik KP, Dehury S, Patro S, Mohanty P, Sahoo SS, et al. Cutaneous adverse drug reactions with fixed-dose combinations: Special reference to self-medication and preventability. Indian J Pharmacol. 2018 ;50(4):192-6.

35. Gupta YK, Ramachandran SS. Fixed dose drug combinations: Issues and challenges in India. Indian J Pharmacol. 2016 ;48(4) :347-9.

36. Chou YJ, Chang HC. Erythema pigmentosum fixans. CMAJ Can Med Assoc J. 15 Nov 2022;194(44): E1520-1.

37. Saka B, Kombaté K, Médougou BH, Akakpo S, Mouhari-Toure A, Boukari T, et al. Fixed erythema pigmentosa in dermatological practice in Lomé (Togo): retrospective study of 321 cases. Bull Société Pathol Exot. 1 Dec 2012 ;105(5) :384-7.

38. Ordoqui E, De Barrio M, Rodríguez VM, Herrero T, Gil PJ, Baeza ML. Cross-sensitivity among oxicams in piroxicam-caused fixed drug eruption: two case reports. Allergy. Sept 1995 ;50(9):741-4.

39. Ben Romdhane H, Ammar H, Ben Fadhel N, Chadli Z, Ben Fredj N, Boughattas NA, et al. Piroxicam-induced fixed drug eruption: Cross-reactivity with meloxicam. Contact Dermatitis. Juill 2019 ;81(1) :24-6.

40. Slim R, Ouni B, Sahnoun D, Ghariani N, Denguezli M, Fathallah N, et al. Fixed erythema pigmentosa induced by non-steroidal anti-inflammatory drugs: experience of the Sousse regional pharmacovigilance centre. Rev Fr Allergol. 1 mai 2021 ;61(4) :281.

41. Sassi W, Hammami H, Khayat O, Ben Brahim E, Zaouak A, Rabhi F, et al. Pristinamycin-induced erythema pigmentum fixans. Ann Dermatol Venereology. May 1, 2018;145(4, Supplement):A50.

42. Vikramjeet S, Angelika B, Nishtha M. Norfloxacin Induced Recurrent Fixed Drug Eruption in a self Treated Adult Female Patient - A Case Report. Curr Drug Saf. 2019 ;14(1):72-6.

43. Sánchez-Morillas L, Rojas Pérez-Ezquerra P, González Morales ML, Mayorga C, González-Mendiola R, Laguna Martínez JJ. Fixed drug eruption due to norfloxacin and cross-reactivity with other quinolones. Allergol Immunopathol (Madr). 2013 ;41(1) :60-1.

44. Kouotou EA, Nansseu JR, Ngono VN, Tatah SA, Zoung-Kanyi Bissek AC, Ndjitoyap Ndam EC. Prevalence and Clinical Profile of Drug Eruptions among Antiretroviral Therapy-Exposed HIV Infected People in Yaoundé, Cameroon. Dermatol Res Pract. 2017 ;2017 :6216193.

45. Sachdeva RK, Sharma A, De D, Malhi J, Rewari BB, Singh S, et al. Lamivudine-Induced Skin Rash Remains an Underdiagnosed Entity in HIV: A Case Series from a Single Center. J Int Assoc Provid AIDS Care. 2016 ;15(2) :153-8.

46. Walmsley SL, Antela A, Clumeck N, Duiculescu D, Eberhard A, Gutiérrez F, et al. Dolutegravir plus abacavir-lamivudine for the treatment of HIV-1 infection. N Engl J Med. 7 Nov 2013 ;369(19) :1807-18.

47. Bursztejn AC, Rat AC, Tréchot P, Cuny JF, Schmutz JL, Barbaud A. Results of skin tests in the investigation of toxidermia. Ann Dermatol Vénéréologie. 1 Nov 2010 ;137(11) :688-94.

48. Assier H, Valeyrie-Allanore L, Gener G, Verlinde Carvalh M, Chosidow O, Wolkenstein P. Patch testing in non-immediate cutaneous adverse drug reactions: value of extemporaneous patch tests. Contact Dermatitis. 2017 ;77(5) :297-302.

49. Agodokpessi G, Dossou-Yovo S, Hountohotegbe T, Panou M, Djogbessi D, Bigot C, et al. Evaluation of sensitization to 3 common trophallergens in children followed for asthma and/or allergic rhinitis in sub-Saharan Africa: comparative study of prick test and IgE assay in Cotonou, Benin. Rev Fr Allergol. 1 Sep 2018 ;58(5) :361-6.

50. Viarnaud A, Perron E, Chosidow O, Wolkenstein P, Oro S, Ortonne N. Fixed erythema pigmentosum: anatomoclinical analysis of a cohort of 73 patients. Ann Dermatol Venereology. 1 Dec 2017 ;144(12, Supplement): S138.

APPENDICES

DATA COLLECTION FORM

Centre : CUDEV

CMP

Allada N **° file** : ....

Year of consultation: /__/__/__/__/ **Telephone**:....................

1. IDENTITY

Age : /__/__/in years **Sex** : M F

Profession : Civil servant Self-employed (manual worker, craftsman, dressmaker ......) Pupil/Student Business Unemployed

Marital status: Married Common-law Single Divorced Widowed **Department of origin**: Littoral / Atlantique Ouémé / Plateau

Zou / Hills Mono / Couffo Alibori / Borgou Atacora / Donga

Place of residence : Rural Urban

2. REASON FOR CONSULTATION :

Fluid lesions Black spots

Localized pruritus Local pain Others............

3. PERSONAL ANTECEDENTS

Atopy: Asthma Sinusitis Allergic conjunctivitis Allergic rhinitis

Eczema None

HIV serology: yes no If yes, year: /__/__ /__/__/ ART: yes no

Diabetes: yes no If yes, year: /__/__ /__/__ /

HTA: yes no If yes, year: /__/__ /__/__ /

Systemic lupus erythematosus: yes no If yes, year: /__/__ /__/__ /

Hepatopathy: yesno If yes, year: /__/__ /__/__ /

Nephropathy: yesno If yes, year: /__/__ /__/__ /

Rheumatoid arthritis: yes no If yes, year: /__/__ /__/__ /

Sickle cell disease: yes no

Self-medication: yes no

Drug addiction: yes no

Alcoholism: yes no

4. CLINICAL ELEMENTS

Number of episodes : 1er 2(e) 3th >3

Time of occurrence in days: Less than 24 hours

24H - 48H

more than 48 hours

Drugs involved: yes no If yes, please specify:....................

Food in question: yes no If yes, please specify:....................

Medication taken for the first time: yes no If yes, please specify:............

First feeding: yes no If yes, please specify:.............

Time to consultation: /__/__/in terms of days

Route : Home - Hospital

Home - self-medication - hospital

home - traditional practitioner - hospital

Alcohol intake: yes no Quantity: /__/__/in grams

Tobacco use: yes no Quantity: /__/

Illness causing the medication: yes no If yes, please specify:.................

Weight :.......... **Size :........** **Temperature :...... ;**

Seat of lesions : Head

Neck

Thoracic region

Lumbar region

Sacred region

Abdominal region

Thoracic limb

Pelvic limb

EMB

Mucosal damage

General

If mucous membranes are affected, specify: oral

ocular

vaginal

Anal

Type of lesions : Vesicles

Bullous lesions

Black spots

Erythema

Number of lesions: /__/__/ Skin area affected (Wallace): /__/%

Evolution: Favourable

Unfavourable

Complication : Impetiginisation

Eczema

Ulceration

Hyperpigmented sequelae

Deaths

5. **BALANCE SHEET REQUESTS** :

HIV serology: yesno If yes, please specify: positive negative

Fasting blood glucose: yes no If yes, specify: normal high

CBC: yes no If yes, please specify :

Hepatitis serology: yes no If yes, please specify :

Patch test: yes no If yes, type of test: ....

Results: positive negative

Skin biopsy: yes no If yes, please specify

Drug liability: yes no If yes, please specify

Other to be specified: ....

6. **CLINICAL FORM**: Bullous EPF

   General EPF

Non-pigmented EPF

EPF in its common form

7.TREATMENT

Eviction certificate: drawn up presented not seen

Medication: Antiseptic

antibiotics

painkillers

emollients

other to be specified:..................

Appointments Checks yes no

TABLE OF CONTENTS

FSC
www.fsc.org
MIX
Papier | Fördert
gute Waldnutzung
FSC® C083411

Kolibri 360 GmbH
Ferdinand-Jühlke-Straße 7
99095 Erfurt, Deutschland
produktsicherheit@kolibri360.de

Druck:
CPI Druckdienstleistungen GmbH
im Auftrag der
Kolibri 360 GmbH
Ferdinand-Jühlke-Str. 7
99095 Erfurt